T0234504

Top Tips in Anaesthesia

Top Tips in Anaesthesia

Edited by

Dr T M Perris
Consultant Anaesthetist
Gloucester Royal Hospital
UK

Dr C S Brudney
Assistant Clinical Professor
Department of Anaesthesiology
Duke University Medical Center
USA

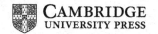
CAMBRIDGE
UNIVERSITY PRESS

CAMBRIDGE
UNIVERSITY PRESS

University Printing House, Cambridge CB2 8BS, United Kingdom

One Liberty Plaza, 20th Floor, New York, NY 10006, USA

477 Williamstown Road, Port Melbourne, VIC 3207, Australia

314-321, 3rd Floor, Plot 3, Splendor Forum, Jasola District Centre, New Delhi - 110025, India

103 Penang Road, #05-06/07, Visioncrest Commercial, Singapore 238467

Cambridge University Press is part of the University of Cambridge.

It furthers the University's mission by disseminating knowledge in the pursuit of
education, learning and research at the highest international levels of excellence.

www.cambridge.org
Information on this title: www.cambridge.org/9781841101712

© Cambridge University Press 2005

A catalogue record for this publication is available from the British Library

ISBN 978-1-841-10171-2 Paperback

....

Every effort has been made in preparing this book to provide accurate and
up-to-date information which is in accord with accepted standards and practice
at the time of publication. Although case histories are drawn from actual cases,
every effort has been made to disguise the identities of the individuals involved.
Nevertheless, the authors, editors and publishers can make no warranties that the
information contained herein is totally free from error, not least because clinical
standards are constantly changing through research and regulation. The authors,
editors and publishers therefore disclaim all liability for direct or consequential
damages resulting from the use of material contained in this book. Readers
are strongly advised to pay careful attention to information provided by the
manufacturer of any drugs or equipment that they plan to use.

CONTENTS

PREFACE

One of the joys of anaesthesia is that there is no "right" way to do it.

There are as many possible permutations to every clinical situation as there are anaesthetists working. That having been said, some ways are more "right" than others and there are definitely lots of "wrong" ways too.

Training and technology have made anaesthesia, for the most part, very safe. However, every practitioner has been in difficulties at some time in their career. If you have not, one has not been doing it long enough!

What we have sought in this collection of "Top Tips" (how to do it) and "Caveats" (how not to do it) is to compile the *pearls of wisdom* that have been passed down from colleagues all around the world. These are the small details of practice that we have come to rely on when the going gets tough. Most of them are too obscure or even down right strange to make the mainstream textbooks. Many are not "evidence based." We are not seeking to rival the Cochrane Database, but do believe that, worthy as that scholarly collection may be, there is still a place in medicine for skill, artistry and individualism. We are merely trying to spread the word slightly further and perhaps add another string to a few bows for those times when the available options seem a little limited.

Some readers may consider parts of the book familiar or basic in the extreme – perhaps because the authors had the same teachers as you. Indeed, some tips are obvious, but we all have to learn from somewhere. We are aiming at both beginners and experts and make no apologies for covering a broad range. It has been a fascinating experience for us, sifting through so many different ideas from practitioners on both sides of the Atlantic and all over the world. We do not necessarily agree with all of them and would encourage a healthy degree of scepticism about anything written here. These are merely suggestions that experienced colleagues have found to be of use in certain challenging situations.

We also do not accept responsibility for the safety or efficacy of the advice. That is down to those who supplied it. We have included the vast majority of tips submitted and trust our readers to evaluate the advice with intelligence and care before trying them on patients.

We make no claims that this is, by any means, an exhaustive or indeed original collection. We have added our names or those of the contributors to each tip but we are certainly not the first to dream them up. We are merely the means by which this collection of "folk wisdom" has been compiled. Anyone who feels they have been stripped of their intellectual property should inform us and we will add your credit to any future edition. While you are at it, send us some more tips and we will include those too.

As we said at the beginning, there are as many techniques as anaesthetists. As a learned colleague expressed it to me, "Anaesthesia is like skinning cats; there are many ways to do it, but few of them are elegant!" We hope you can find at least a few that are useful to your practice.
Good luck

Tom Perris
Consultant Anaesthetist
Gloucester Royal Hospital
UK

C Scott Brudney
Assistant Clinical Professor
Department of Anesthesiology
Duke University Medical Center
USA

AIRWAY MANAGEMENT

AIRWAY MANAGEMENT

One of the key skills of the anaesthetist and one that sets us apart from most of our fellow doctors is the ability to maintain and manage the airway. In the vast majority of cases, this is possible with only the simplest of techniques. For the exceptions to this rule, it helps to have a few tricks up your sleeve.

Emergency cricothyroidotomy

The last resort in the "cannot intubate/cannot ventilate" situation is the emergency cricothyroidoty.

A 14-G cannula inserted via the cricothyroid membrane can provide oxygenation (although probably not adequate ventilation). In a hurry – and you will be – it is worth knowing a technique to connect your cannula to the oxygen (O_2) supply.

Tip

1. A standard connector from a size 7.0 COETT will fit into the barrel of a 2 mL syringe. The syringe will attach to the cannula; the connector can be attached to a self-inflating bag.
2. The barrel of a 1 mL syringe with the flanges snapped off can be forced into O_2 tubing from a wall-mounted supply. A hole can be made by snipping across a corner of a kink in the tubing. By intermittently occluding the hole with your thumb, an on–off effect can be achieved.
3. Attach a 10 mL syringe (with the barrel removed) to your cannula, then insert your endotracheal (ET) tube into this and blow up the cuff.

Caveat

The pressure from a wall outlet is 4 bar – quite enough to cause severe barotrauma. Usually, but not always, the patient can exhale. Watch for breath stacking. Lean on the chest (gently!) to assist exhalation.

Tom Perris, Gloucester, UK

Nasotracheal intubation

To facilitate surgical access to the mouth and oropharynx or to prevent the patient biting down and occluding the ET tube, nasal intubation can be employed.

However, it is not without its drawbacks:

- Epistaxis can be severe or even fatal in the presence of a coagulopathy.
- Trauma to the nasal passages is frequent.
- Tubes can cause pressure necrosis to the nares, particularly if left *in situ* for extended periods.
- Ventilation acquired pneumonia (VAP) increases significantly with nasal intubation.

Tip

Prepare the nose with vasoconstrictor. Cocaine has the twin benefits of limiting bleeding and providing local anaesthesia. Do not exceed the safe dose (approximately 150 mg in adults).

Check which nostril is most patent either with a "sniff" test or, after the patient is asleep, with a gloved finger gently inserted into the nostril.

The nasal passage runs directly posterior, perpendicular to the face not upwards.

Gently insert the tube using the chosen nostril. If the tube does not "turn the corner" and enter the oropharynx, it can be guided around the soft palate with a finger in the mouth helping it. Do not force it! The posterior pharyngeal wall can be damaged.

Do not cut your tube; let it dangle to prevent pressure sores caused by the connector.

Tom Perris, Gloucester, UK

Paediatric intubation

The paediatric larynx differs from the adult in several important ways:

- It is smaller, higher and more anterior than the adult.
- It is more funnel shaped.
- The narrowest part is the cricoid ring not the vocal cords.
- The epiglottis is relatively large and floppy.

This can lead to difficulties during intubation.

Tip

Choose the correct size of tube.

A rotatory movement can alleviate difficulty in inserting the tube past the cords or cricoid.

During nasal intubation in children (and, to a lesser extent, adults) the ET tube approaches the larynx from a posterior position. The larynx and trachea descend from anterior to posterior, so an angle exists between tube and trachea that can cause obstruction below the cords.

The remedy is, once the tube is positioned, release the pressure of the hand performing laryngoscopy, so the larynx drops out of sight. This straightens the angle and allows the tube to pass easily.

Fiona Reynolds, Birmingham Children's Hospital, UK

Difficult intubation

Intubation is usually simple ... but not always!

Tip

In a difficulty to intubate/ventilate patient, place two nasopharyngeal airways and attach the connector from an ET tube. Ventilate at high-tidal volumes and a high rate. Usually you can ventilate easily.

Ellen Flannagan, Duke, USA

Tip

If a patient can be ventilated and not intubated and ear, nose and throat (ENT) surgeons are around they can often position an ET tube with a rigid bronchoscope!

Paddy McNight, Whipps Cross, London

Tip

In all matters concerning anaesthesia but particularly with potential difficult airways, have a plan B (and plan C). Tell your assistant what they are.

Alison Wright, Warwick, UK

Tip

Positioning is everything.

To ensure optimal intubating conditions, align the ear with the sternal notch (in the horizontal plane). This is especially important in the obese or those with long necks. You may need extra pillows.

If you are using a stylette, shape it straight to the cuff and only angle the tip. More curvature obscures the view.

Alison Wright, Warwick, UK

Tip

With a probable tricky intubation, never do anything you cannot get out of.

Do not induce till you have preoxygenated fully. Do not stop the patient breathing until you know you can hand ventilate. Do not let the surgeon start until you are completely happy with your airway and do not extubate the patient until you are completely happy that they have it back under their own control.

Tom Perris, Gloucester, UK

Tip

Do not be tempted to extubate the patient too early.

No one ever died from keeping their tube for an extra minute but lots have from taking it out before full recovery.

Gary Levin, San Francisco, USA

Tip

When confronted with a Grade 3 intubation, bend the tip of a gum-elastic bougie to 90°. Run it along the underside of the epiglottis until the corrugations of the trachea can be felt. Railroad the ET tube over the top.

Jim Watt, Birmingham, UK

Tip

Use a nasal airway preferentially at induction. If the attempt at intubation should fail, you already have an airway *in situ*, reducing the likelihood of desaturation.

Lewis R Hodgins, Duke, USA

AIRWAY MANAGEMENT
Fibreoptic intubation

Tip

In the patient with a larynx sited more anterior than usual, do not hyper-extend the neck during intubation or place a sandbag under the shoulders. Rather, flex the head, releasing the strap muscles. This will allow the larynx to be displaced backwards using cricoid pressure. Hopefully your view will improve.

Lewis R Hodgins, Duke, USA

Tip

Use the intubating laryngeal mask airway (LMA) early. Rather than struggling with conventional tools, reach for the LMA Fastrach. This provides a rapid airway. If the ET tube does not advance easily, a bronchoscope can be used to check for the seating of the LMA.

Scott Brudney, Duke, USA

Fibreoptic intubation

Tip

If a fibreoptic scope is not available, or provides a poor view, use an adult scope and pass a 0.97 mm ×150 cm guide-wire down the port. This can then be used as a guide-wire to thread an ET tube over.

Ian Welsby, Duke, USA

Tip

For rapid awake fibreoptic intubation (FOI), make the patient sit up to 45°. Administer aliquots of fentanyl *only* for sedation. This keeps the patient responsive. Start by using xylocaine 10% spray, only enough to obtain access to the mouth. Using an atomiser mist the back of the throat and oropharynx with 4% lignocaine; 2–4 mL will give excellent anaesthesia.

Insert an intubating airway, place a size 6.0 COETT over the scope, attach high flow O_2 to the suction port (this will help oxygenate and blow debris out the way), then advance the scope through the airway. When the epiglottis and cords are visualised, inject 2×2 mL 4% lignocaine, allow to settle and then advance the scope. Once through the cords administer some propofol and then advance the tube.

Scott Brudney, Duke, USA

Microlaryngoscopy and laser therapy to vocal cords

It is always a challenge sharing an airway with a surgeon, particularly if they need to undertake potentially hazardous laser procedures around the larynx. To protect against airway fires, various non-combustible tubes have been developed. These, however, are bulky and obscure the surgeons' view. Several techniques have been employed to surmount these difficulties. This is an elegant one.

Caveat

This is not a technique for a patient gasping with stridor – an inhalational induction would be my technique of choice in that situation.

Tip

Induce with propofol 2 mg/kg followed by infusion of 12 mg/kg/h.

Draw 1 mg alfentanil up to 10 mL. Give 70 µg/kg to start (half an ampoule approximately). Mask ventilate with 100% O_2.

Have 5 mL of 2% lignocaine for intravenous (i.v.) use drawn up.

At laryngoscopy, generously spray the epiglottic fold, vocal cords and arytenoids with the lignocaine you have just drawn up. Make sure lots go through into the trachea. I attach a blue needle to the syringe with it bent 45° and use this.

The i.v. lignocaine is the trick, so they do not cough.

Do not use the lignocaine spray. It is dissolved in 90% alcohol and is extremely irritating.

Mask ventilate for another 30–60 s with 100% O_2.

Allow the surgeon to insert the rigid laryngoscope. Even if the patient is still apnoeic they will stay saturated because of the preoxygenation.

I find that with the lignocaine the stimulus is gentle enough that they start breathing and not bucking.

Once they breathe, titrate small aliquots of alfentanil – hence the dilution to 10 mL.

If they breathe well, the patient will actually maintain saturation on room air allowing the surgeon an uninterrupted, unobstructed view.

Sometimes it is necessary to dribble in a little extra O_2. Just take your circuit of choice, dial in O_2 and room air till you have 40% (3 L air + 1 L O_2 approximately) and let it flow into the mouth and rigid scope.

When finished – Guedel airway, non-steroidal anti-inflammatory drug (NSAID) of choice +/− opioid.

Just one more point: they must not have a cold!!! The airways are too reactive and they just cough.

Blaine Robson, Port Elizabeth, South Africa

Single lung ventilation

Tip

If you use a "univent" tube for one lung intubation, the following helps direct the blocker into the desired bronchus:

Use the usual Magill blade for intubation. Advance the tube through the larynx with the curvature of the tube at 12 o'clock. With the laryngoscope still in the mouth, rotate the tube to the 3 o'clock position if you want to block the right lung, 9 o'clock if it is left you are after. Advance the blocker prior to removing the laryngoscope.

The "traditional" method of moving the head in the opposite direction has caused me difficulties. The above modification has resulted in correct blocking every time.

Sugantha Ganapathy, Duke, USA

Tip

Having trouble positioning your double lumen tube? Get the surgeons to do it! It is in their best interests to have it properly placed!

Scott Brudney, Duke, USA

Be nice to your patients ...

Always give good advice, however much you may feel otherwise!

> **Tip**
>
> Warm the plastic nasal tube in hot water to soften it before use. It will cause less trauma to the nasal passage and turn the corner more easily.
>
> *Jim Watt, Birmingham, UK*

> **Tip**
>
> Use lignocaine gel on the ET to decrease sore throat/coughing on extubation.
>
> *Jonathan Chantler, Oxford, UK*

Mask seal for bearded or edentulous patients

The authors are against facial hair for several reasons: not least because it makes face mask ventilation difficult.

> **Tip**
>
> A satisfactory mask seal is often difficult to obtain in bearded or edentulous patients. A moistened, large combine pad with a hole cut for ventilation in the centre may help provide a good seal.
>
> The mask, water, skin interfaces are airtight at usual airway pressures during spontaneous and assisted ventilation with or without positive end expiratory pressure (PEEP).
>
> *Joel S Goldberg, North Carolina, USA*

Flexible laryngeal mask insertion

The LMA (LMA-Flexible™) is a useful device to guard against surgical interference with the airway. It is, however, notoriously tricky to insert. This may help.

Tip

Carry a size six uncut, paediatric oral ET tube in your bag, for use with armoured LMAs. Lightly lubricate the ET tube and then insert into the lumen of the LMA. It acts as a splint and makes the insertion as simple as a normal LMA.

Remember to remove the ET tube before you connect up the circuit!

Malcolm Savidge, Gloucester, UK

Tip

Magill's forceps can be used to insert an armoured LMA. Grip it at the junction of cuff and tube. Gently guide the LMA around the side of the tongue and push it down into the pharynx. This saves getting spit on your fingers or being bitten if the patient's light!

Tom Perris, Gloucester, UK

Tip

Swap positions with your operating department assistant (ODA)/practitioner/resident/nurse anaesthetist and insert the LMA from in front of the patient. The LMA will advance much more easily than from the head end.

Scott Brudney, Duke, USA

Inadvertent damage to the pilot tube

Occasionally, the pilot tube can be accidentally cut. If, at this time, changing the tube would be against the patient's best interests, this is an ingenious holding measure.

Tip

Insert two 18-G blunt needles (drawing-up needles) into each end of the cut pilot tube. They fit snugly. Join the two with a male-to-male i.v. connector. It should now be possible to re-inflate the cuff.

Gary Levin, San Francisco, USA

2

PREOPERATIVE ASSESSMENT AND OPTIMISATION

Warning signs

Forewarned is forearmed. Having an idea that your patient may be less than healthy allows you to formulate a plan at leisure rather than rethinking your entire anaesthetic in times of crisis.

You might want to watch out for the following.

Left bundle branch block

Tip

Beware of the patient with left bundle branch block (LBBB) on their preoperative electrocardiograph (ECG). Because it obscures the true shape of the ST segment, we tend to forget that it represents a potentially severe degree of ischaemic heart disease.

Development of LBBB during anaesthesia similarly implies myocardial hypoperfusion.

Treat promptly as for angina. I like to get the blood pressure (BP) up and the pulse rate down. Metaraminol usually works for this +/− beta blocker of choice (if not contraindicated).

Tom Perris, Gloucester, UK

Metabolic acidosis

Tip

Any patient with a base deficit of four or greater requires review by a senior clinician.

Julian Bion, Birmingham, UK

Raised respiratory rate

> **Tip**
>
> The respiratory rate is often the earliest and most sensitive sign of a deteriorating physiological state and an unwell patient.
>
> Beware of anyone who appears to be working too hard at his or her breathing.
>
> Elucidation of the cause and, if possible, remedial action should be undertaken prior to anaesthesia.
>
> *Tom Perris, Gloucester, UK*

Optimisation goals

We would all wish to have our patients in the best possible condition prior to surgery. Preoptimisation has been proven to improve outcome. Having an endpoint to aim for allows you to judge the adequacy of your intervention.

Preoperative admission to intensive care and invasive monitoring may be required.

> **Tip**
>
> All "high risk" patients having a general anaesthetic should be resuscitated until their mixed venous saturation (SVO_2) exceeds 70%.
>
> *Julian Bion, Birmingham, UK*

When in doubt ....

Tip

The answer is "volume".

Lewis R Hodgins, Duke, USA

Likewise ....

Tip

Dialysis patients are generally hypovolaemic.

Lewis R Hodgins, Duke, USA

Tip

Anyone who has had bowel preparation is not only hypovolaemic but also hypokalaemic too. It is worth checking a blood gas prior to induction or very soon afterwards.

Tom Perris, Gloucester, UK

Obesity

Sadly, becoming more common.

Many potential problems arise for the anaesthetist with obese patients. Raised intra-abdominal pressure is one of them. When deciding on your technique, consider this ....

Tip

When supine, if the apex of the patient's abdomen is higher than the tip of their nose, a laryngeal mask airway (LMA) is a poor choice.

Jo Cobbe, Gloucester, UK

Tip

To prevent the arms falling off the table when inducing an obese patient, ask them to clasp their hands together, for some reason they will stay clasped post-induction!

Ian Crabb, Gloucester, UK

Tip

Patient too large for the operating table? Tie two tables together!

Scott Brudney, Duke, USA

Tip

Always have a short handled laryngoscope on hand.

Too big for non-invasive BP (even on calf or forearm)? Site an arterial line with the help of a doppler.

Despite regional being a daunting task it is worth attempting a block. They are frequently easier than one at first imagines and well worth it if general anaesthesia (GA) can be avoided.

Scott Brudney, Duke, USA

3

PRACTICAL PROCEDURES AND TECHNIQUES

Central venous catheter placement

The uses of central venous cannulation are many and varied. They include vascular access for inotropes and other potent or irritant drugs, total parenteral nutrition (TPN), dialysis, measurement of central pressures, cardiac catheterisation/biopsy, insertion of pulmonary artery (PA) catheters and pacing wires are all feasible via a central vein.

In an attempt to reduce the potentially serious complications associated with the use of central venous catheter placement (CVP) lines, recent guidance from the National Institute of Clinical Excellence (NICE, UK) recommends the use of ultrasound to assist with placement.

Where this is available, we would support its use. However, most of us were trained prior to the advent of such aids. We include a few tips learned over the years.

PRACTICAL PROCEDURES AND TECHNIQUES
Central venous catheter placement

Tip

Examine the neck for venous pulsation. Insert needle at the midpoint of the pulsation.

If the patient is conscious, get them to perform a Valsalva manoeuvre. It considerably increases the cross-sectional area of the vein.

If the patient is intubated, an inspiratory hold will perform the same function. So will an increase in positive end-expiratory pressure (PEEP) or plateau pressure.

Lewis Hodgins, Duke, USA

Caveat

This may be detrimental in some patients, particularly those with low cardiac output and/or hypovolaemia.

Tom Perris, Gloucester, UK

Tip

Transduction of central lines increases the certainty of correct venous placement. This technique is quick and easy.

After opening your CVP pack, attach a three-way stopcock to the end of your large-bore needle. Connect the syringe to one port, a sterile pressure transducer tubing set to the other and flush all air out.

Find what you believe to be the vein as normal. Turn the stopcock to open the pressure transducer and observe the trace. If it is venous you will see a CVP waveform. If it is arterial, the typical tracing will be seen. If correct placement is confirmed, open the stopcock to the needle and insert the guide-wire. Remove syringe, stopcock and needle as one unit leaving the guide-wire. With this method you can avoid embarrassing and dangerous dilatation of a large artery.

Aaron Ali, Duke, USA

Tip

When performing an invasive procedure, such as central venous cannulation, line the bevel of the needle up with the numbers on the syringe barrel. This way, you can tell the orientation of the needle no matter how deeply it is inserted.

Allan B Shang, Duke, USA

Tip

Compress the IJV with a finger and briskly release the pressure. Careful observation of the neck shows the vein re-filling. This allows a pretty good visualisation of the position of the vein.

Tom Perris, Gloucester, UK

Tip

I always use the plastic cannula supplied in the central line pack rather than the large-bore steel needle. It is easy to use and offers several advantages:

- It can safely be left inside the vein whilst attempting to thread the Seldinger wire. The sharp metal needle risks lacerating the vein whilst you reach for the wire.
- You can confirm placement inside the vein by aspiration of venous blood at any time or even transduce the pressure if unsure.
- Whilst I do not recommend resheathing needles, after the first guide-wire is in place, you can (carefully) re-use the cannula to insert a second access port into the IJV. Simply find the vein as before (the wire will give you a marker) and leave the cannula in the vein. Secure it, later, with a dressing.
- If a PA sheath, PA catheter or haemofiltration line is required later, you now have ready access to the central veins for a guide-wire without risking lacerating the existing CVP line with a sharp needle in the same vein.

Tom Perris, Gloucester, UK

Tip

When attempting to insert a subclavian CVP line in a dehydrated patient, make sure the bevel of your needle faces the feet to maximise flashback.

Alison Wright, Warwick, UK

Tip

Use full monitoring when inserting your lines. A burst of ventricular ectopics confirms placement and warns you to pull back your guide-wire a little.

Sudden desaturation or loss of carbon dioxide (CO_2) trace suggests a possible tension pneumothorax.

Tom Perris, Gloucester, UK

Tip

When palpating the neck to ascertain the position of the carotid artery prior to attempting an IJV line, make sure you release the pressure before you cannulate. The vein will be squashed flat by your fingers if you keep pushing. Lifting the jaw with your other hand may, conversely, open the vein wider.

Scott Brudney, Duke, USA

Arterial line insertion

Arterial access has many advantages. It gives you real-time, beat-to-beat variation in blood pressure (BP). It allows rapid blood sampling for measurement of gases and electrolytes and by visualisation of the waveform, an assessment of the patient's haemodynamics can be made.

Inserting an arterial line, however, can be one of the most frustrating activities known to man. Also, it is not pleasant for the patient.

Hope this helps.

Tip

Do not overextend the wrist. It occludes the pulse.

Alison Wright, Warwick, UK

Tip

Approach the vessel at a shallow angle. It improves your chances of entering it. If you hit bone, pull back, decrease the angle and try again. If you are wearing gloves, the vessel seems often to be more medial than the pulse you feel.

Sock Huang Koh, Birmingham, UK

Tip

A little judicious ephedrine before you start helps correct placement, I find.

I also use local anaesthetic, which not only improves the experience for the patient, but limits vaso-spasm. Rub the area to disperse swelling and restore the anatomy after injection.

Tom Perris, Gloucester, UK

Doppler location of impalpable arteries

Obesity, oedematous limbs, low BP or distorted anatomy can make a tricky job even harder. If you suspect that you are going to encounter difficulties when attempting arterial puncture, try the following idea.

Tip

Using a suitable lubricant, place a Doppler probe at the expected site of the chosen vessel. Locate the best signal of pulsatile flow and aim your cannula at this area. Keep the volume turned up. As the needle approaches the artery, the signal can be used to guide your way. It takes a little practice but usually works quite reliably.

Ben Walton, Bristol, UK

The most serious complication of arterial cannulation, though uncommon, is potentially devastating. Thrombosis of an end-vessel can cause ischaemic damage to the entire limb necessitating amputation.

Allen's test was traditionally used to assess the adequacy of the ulnar collateral circulation prior to radial artery cannulation. Both pulses are occluded by direct pressure whilst the patient clenches the fist to cause blanching of the skin. Upon release of the ulnar pressure, the colour should return briskly to the palm within 5–10 s. Longer time implies a deficient ulnar circulation.

Unfortunately, Allen's test has proved unreliable and is unfeasible in the anaesthetised patient in theatre or intensive care unit (ICU).

The pulse oximeter is, not only, excellent at measuring oxygen (O_2) saturation of arterial blood. It is also exquisitely sensitive in detecting pulsation. It can be used to assess the quality of the ulnar collateral circulation.

Tip

Place the sats' probe on a finger as normal. Occlude the ulnar and radial arteries with pressure to the wrist. Release the pressure of each in turn (ulnar first). A good Sats' trace when the ulnar circulation is restored suggests an adequate blood supply from that side.

Scott Brudney, Duke, USA

PA catheterisation

Lack of proven benefit and increasing use of alternative monitoring modalities seems to be leading to a reduction in the use of PA catheters. They do, however, still have their uses and advocates.

PA catheters carry with them the disadvantages and potential complications of all major vascular access procedures plus a few all of their own. Vascular or cardiac damage, arrhythmias, infection/endocarditis and pulmonary infarction are all recorded complications.

On the positive side, a wealth of useful information can be obtained:

Mixed venous, right atrial, and ventricular gas tensions and saturations can be measured and shunt calculations can be performed. Direct measurement of the PA pressure, capillary wedge pressure and cardiac output plus calculation of systemic and pulmonary vascular resistances can be of use in patients with compromised circulation.

Like with many invasive procedures, the more you need one, the harder it is to put in.

We include a few tips.

Tip

If excessive resistance is encountered while passing a PA catheter through an introducer, apply counter traction or withdraw the introducer sheath a centimetre or so. The end of the sheath may be up against a vessel wall preventing passage of the catheter.

Lewis R Hodgins, Duke, USA

Tip

If the PA catheter has lost its rigidity after several unsuccessful attempts to float it, try flushing it with ice-cold saline.

Jonathan Chantler, Oxford, UK

The distal tip of a PA catheter is frequently aligned in the 11 or 12 o'clock position before inserting into the introducer sheath. This may facilitate floatation of the catheter into the proper position. After insertion, the catheter can get twister losing proper alignment. A method to maintain and reference the tip position using a proximal port at the 30 cm mark is described.

Tip

Hold the catheter, partially curled, in one hand.

With slight tension on the catheter, hold it in the 12 o'clock position with respect to the introducer

Look down the axis of the catheter. The "clock" position of a proximal port is noted. (Imagine a cross section of the catheter at 30 cm to represent the face of a clock, which is aligned to the introducer sheath.) The numerical position of the port is used as a reference mark.

The catheter is now inserted beginning with the tip positioned at 12 o'clock. At 30 cm, the position of the proximal port is noted.

The catheter can be twisted to return the tip to the ideal 12 o'clock position if it has rotated during insertion. This hopefully assists correct placement.

Joel S Goldberg, Duke, USA

Which approach?

For ease of insertion of a PA catheter, I would choose the left subclavian approach.

▼

The curve into the innominate vein and onwards into the superior vena cava is smooth. From the right subclavian, a sharp turn has to be executed.

Similarly, the path from the right internal jugular vein is straighter than from the left.

Tom Perris, Gloucester, UK

Early warning sign for cardiac ischaemia

Tip

The papillary muscles that control mitral and tricuspid valve closure are situated within the ventricle and thus are furthest from the coronary arterial supply. Consequently they are vulnerable to ischaemia.

With a PA catheter is *in situ*, new onset mitral regurgitation (seen as giant V waves on the PA trace) or tricuspid regurgitation (seen on the CVP waveform) may be an early sign of myocardial hypo-perfusion.

Caveat

If you watch the CVP waveform whilst volume loading, as the heart becomes full, tricuspid regurgitation is frequently seen. This is not necessarily due to ischaemia, but simple mechanical distension of the atrium causing a leak through the valve.

It is a good idea to slow your intravenous (i.v.) infusion down at this point!

Tom Perris, Gloucester, UK

Transoesophageal echocardiography (TOE/TEE)

Transesophageal echocardiography (TEE) under general anaesthesia is facilitated by the use of small tidal volumes and increased respiratory rates. This will reduce the tidal movement of structures during examination.

Lewis R Hodgins, Duke, USA

Be nice

Tip

Warm your Lignocaine (Lidocaine) in your pocket whilst setting up for procedures. It stings less that way.

Jonathan Chantler, Oxford, UK.

Tip

When inserting a large-bore i.v. cannula, use local anaesthetic.

To inject the local, use a 25-G needle with the bevel facing downwards (i.e. upside-down). This reduces the pain of injection for the patient.

Chris Roberts, Gloucester, UK

Difficult spinal

Tip

When inserting a spinal, remember, the patient is the best source of information.

If landmarks are hard to come by, try asking the patient where he feels the needle, "Left, right or in the middle."

Sometimes, where the needle is felt and where you think it should be, are not the same at all. The patient is usually correct.

Scott Brudney, Duke, USA

Spinals in the elderly

Tip

When using Heavy Marcaine in a patient in the lateral position, (e.g. a patient with fractured neck of femur) it is worthwhile having a head-up tilt on the table or by placing pillows beneath the head and shoulders. This prevents rapid cephalic spread of the Marcaine and ensures a low block with minimal hypotension.

When you are putting such a patient on the table and the automatic BP has yet to record the pressure, you worry about hypotension.

PRACTICAL PROCEDURES AND TECHNIQUES
Difficult spinal/Spinals in the elderly

If the O_2 saturation monitor is reading low despite apparently adequate respiratory function and supplemental O_2, the most likely cause is hypotension resulting in V/Q mismatch.

I would suggest a prophylactic dose of ephedrine (or an alpha agonist depending on pulse rate) whilst waiting for the BP to finish measuring.

Scott Brudney, Duke, USA

Epidurals

Tip

With all practical procedures, but particularly with epidural insertion, there are two things that are paramount.

1. Know your anatomy and do not put anything sharp anywhere unless you know where it is going. If you are not sure where is the tip of your needle, pull it out, reassess and start again.
2. Have all your equipment immediately to hand. Make sure it all works and is correctly assembled. Halfway through an epidural or CVP line insertion is not the time to be reaching across and trying to draw up saline, flush the catheter or whatever. Get it ready before you start.

Tom Perris, Gloucester, UK

Tip

When getting ready for an epidural, aspirate your saline into a normal syringe then squirt it into the loss of resistance device. It is a lot quicker than trying to draw it up with the loss of resistance (LOR) syringe itself, as it does not hold a vacuum.

Alternatively, pour sterile saline into the small pot included in most sets and draw it up from there. Seems to work without a needle.

Jonathan Chantler, Oxford, UK

Tip

Trouble removing the epidural catheter on the ward? Try placing the patient in the same position originally used for the epidural insertion. Never failed yet!

Tony Roche, UK

Tip

If you find difficulty passing the catheter past the end of the Touhy needle, rotate the needle through 180° and try again.

Jim Watt, Birmingham, UK

Regional anaesthetic techniques

Tip

Never force a patient who is unwilling to have a regional block. It will not work.

Also, never be tempted to cover the slight inadequacies of your block with Midazolam.

Better to block the offending missed segment again at a different point or do a proper general anaesthetic (GA).

Ben Walton, Bristol, UK

Interscalene block

Of all the techniques of regional anaesthesia, the interscalene approach to the brachial plexus is perhaps the most hazardous. The concentration of important structures within a small area at the base of the neck means that, more than ever, it is vital to have a sound anatomical knowledge.

Some "collateral damage" nearly always occurs due to the proximity of structures. The phrenic nerve is immediately anterior and is often included in the nerves blocked. For this reason, bilateral interscalene blocks should not be performed, particularly in patients with decreased respiratory reserve. The sympathetic chain also is not far away and a Horner's syndrome is sometimes seen.

The vertebral artery is just deep to your needle running into the circle of Willis. Do not inject into that unless you are really keen to see what local anaesthetic toxicity looks like!

The spinal nerve roots complete with dural cuff are close too. Again, a total spinal is probably not what you are trying to achieve so a thorough grounding in anatomy is essential. Do not go too deep.

The lung is just below you!

Tip

If, in a patient for interscalene block, you cannot feel the groove due to obesity, you can try this.

Ask the patient to lift their head off the pillow. This accentuates the sternomastoid muscle. Put your finger between the two heads and allow the patient to relax back onto the pillow. Walk your finger laterally and your finger comes to rest on the belly of scalenus anterior. Again walk laterally until your finger finds the interscalene groove. Run up the neck until you are at the level of the cricoid.

Failing this, get a Doppler probe to spot the supra-clavicular subclavian artery. Feel the groove behind it and follow it up to the C6 level of the cricoid.

Sugantha Ganapathy, Duke, USA

Tip

i.v. access and full monitoring.

Keep the patient awake so they can assist you. A little sedation is OK but they have to be able to converse with you.

Locate the interscalene groove by palpation. It can be accentuated by getting the patient to sniff deeply and/or lift the head off the pillow.

Mark off the groove with a pen and drop a perpendicular line from the cricoid cartilage. Do not be tempted to follow the skin creases around. You will end up too high in the neck. Mark the intersection.

Local to the skin at the point of insertion and spray or paint with antiseptic of choice.

I use a nerve stimulator set to 0.7 mA. Anything higher is painful and alarming to the patient. Warn them that their arm will start to jump around. A 50 mm "Stimuplex" needle is more than adequate length even in the most obese subjects.

Draw up 30–40 mL of local. (Depends on the size of the patient, type of procedure, etc. but as a rule, 30 mL of 0.375% levobupivacaine works well.)

Do not connect your syringe to the needle, but remove the cap from the injection port. This allows any blood vessel (particularly the vertebral artery) to makes its presence known if you pass into it.

Ensure you have a circuit, (Make sure the light comes on when you touch the skin) and aiming medial, anterior and caudal, carefully advance the needle through the skin. Do not aim perpendicular as it increases the chances of passing between the transverse processes and damaging the vertebral artery. If you hit bone, then you are both too deep and too posterior. You are also dangerously near the vertebral artery.

It may just be me, but I find that I need to aim more anterior than the textbook says. Anyhow, at about 1 cm something will usually begin twitching. If it is deltoid, biceps or pectoralis, you're on the spot. If it is trapezius, you are posterior on the 11th cranial nerve. Realign anterior. If the diaphragm is twitching, you are too anterior.

Even in the biggest people, the plexus is only 1–2 cm deep to the skin. Do not be tempted to go any deeper.... Its Tiger Country in there!

This is where it is useful to have the patient awake. Ask them if what's moving is "neck" (trapezius) or "arm" as it can be difficult to differentiate in the obese when everything wobbles.

Reduce the current to about 0.3 mA. This is the threshold you need for a successful block. If you are finding it difficult to get a reliable twitch at 0.5 mA or less, try advancing your needle a millimetre or two. Sometimes a click is felt as the needle enters the pre-vertebral fascia and the twitch gets stronger. A little time spent getting the exact spot pays dividends here.

Attach your syringe. Aspirate very gently and carefully and inject a test dose of 0.5 mL. It should abolish the twitches and not be painful.

If all is well, continue injecting the rest of the 30–40 mL. Take it steady and warn the patient that it will ache a bit for a while. As the local begins to work, the pain diminishes. A "sausage" of local should be palpable in the neck as it fills the sheath.

If you do not rush to induce general anaesthesia, the patient may experience a reassuring warmth and paraesthesia, indicating successful block.

Caveat

Do not do this block in anyone who could not tolerate even a small pneumothorax or is already at his or her respiratory limit. You will block the phrenic and lose ventilation to some extent.

Watch your safe dose limits on bupivacaine. A decent volume is needed but you can get cardiovascular symptoms if you are near the higher dose limit. Maintain monitoring and be vigilant.

Tom Perris, Gloucester, UK

Axillary block

Jim Watt has, (he is reluctant to inform me,) been providing regional anaesthesia for two hand-surgery lists a week for the last 25 years. He reckons that he has his technique nearly sorted by now. This is his way of doing it.

Tip

Site i.v. access in the other hand. Monitoring *in situ*. Keep the patient awake if you can persuade them.

Put a little local into the skin overlying the axillary pulsation, as you will be taking a little time to locate the nerves.

Asepsis, etc.

Use a 50 mm "Stimuplex" and set your nerve stimulator to 0.4 mA. Any higher risks pain and loss of faith from the patient.

At the level of insertion of the Pectoralis major, palpate the artery and keeping the arm perpendicular in all directions aim just above the artery.

You are aiming for individual nerves at this level. Techniques that rely on spread within the sheath are unreliable. The nerves are, fortunately, arranged in a fairly constant relationship to the artery and with a little practice can be picked off, one by one, quite quickly.

Decide which nerves you will need to block. For palmar surgery, the radial and musculocutaneous are not so vital whereas, if you are using your block for a dialysis fistula or bony surgery, all of the terminal branches may need to be blocked.

The median nerve is large and easy to locate, lying immediately above the artery.

The musculocutaneous (MC) nerve is a little superior to the median. Successful location can be seen with the characteristic twitch. Biceps twitch/supination for the MC, Thumb and lateral fingers flexion for the median. 10 to 12 mL of local is adequate for the median. Five mL or so for the MC.

The radial nerve is below and posterior to the artery. Dorsiflexion of the wrist is the sign you're looking for. Ten mL will effectively block it. Make a new skin puncture about a centimetre below the previous site.

The ulnar nerve is small and more variable in its position but is usually more inferior and superficial than the radial. Medial finger flexion and adduction of the thumb is the sign confirming location.

All these nerves can be reliably located around the elbow if you cannot find them in the axilla. A top-up block can be used if there is no change in sensation after 10 min.

Place the tourniquet as low as possible on the upper arm (but above the ulnar nerve at the elbow) for hand surgery. The anaesthetised portion of the arm is then below the cuff.

Choose your local anaesthetic depending on the type of surgery. Lidocaine is shorter acting but quick; bupivacaine or ropivacaine are slower but longer acting.

Jim Watt, Birmingham, UK

Femoral nerve block

Tip

For this to work properly you need the "Sign of the Dancing Patella" i.e. quadriceps contraction. What you usually get first is medial adductor muscles twitching. Try withdrawing your needle and re-entering the skin a couple of millimetres lateral and perhaps a fraction deeper.

Thirty millilitres of local injected with a finger placed distally pressing down will encourage spread upwards into the femoral plexus.

Consider inserting a femoral sheath catheter if the post-operative pain is going to persist beyond the duration of a single shot. (e.g. a total knee replacement.) You get superior analgaesia and less opiod usage with a dilute infusion of local.

Tom Perris, Gloucester, UK

Biers block

Precision with technique improves efficacy and safety. Again, this is modified with the wisdom of long experience.

Tip

Site i.v. access (for safety) in the opposite hand. Full monitoring *in situ*.

In the hand to be blocked, site a 22-G cannula in retrograde direction. This ensures the site of injection is as distal as possible.

Use an Esmarch bandage to exsanguinate the limb. Do not dislodge the cannula.

Inflate the lower, then the upper cuff of a double tourniquet. 250 mmHg is enough. Let the bottom cuff down again.

Unwind the bandage from the fingers until it is proximal to the site of surgery but still restricts the flow of local up the arm. If you are using this block for carpal tunnel decompression, e.g. unwind the Esmarch to the wrist.

Bend the fingers of the hand downwards to stretch the skin on the dorsum of the hand to encourage spread of local to the palmar side.

Using 0.75% Prilocaine (it is safer and quicker than lidocaine or ropivacaine. Do not use bupivacaine for Biers block) inject 40 mL. Warn the patient it will sting like crazy for a few seconds!

Massage the local around the hand till it covers the area you are trying to block. This stings too.

Unwind the Esmarch and then reapply it from the fingers upwards, spreading the local upwards under the lower cuff. This also limits oozing from the site of surgery. Inflate the lower cuff, which now has local under it making the arm numb. Check whether its up and release the top cuff.

Pinprick test the area of surgery. If it is numb, start. If not, you can top up with another 20 mL. Ensure your cuff pressure is adequate before toping up.

Wait 20 min before releasing the tourniquet. Usually the surgery plus preparation time is over this limit. Release the pressure gradually to avoid a surge in blood level of prilocaine not fixed in the tissues.

For Colles' fracture patients, do not use the Esmarch. It hurts too much. Raise the arm, compress the brachial artery and massage blood from the forearm before you inflate the tourniquet.

Jim Watt, Birmingham, UK

Caveat

Beware of morbidly obese people. However high you set the cuff pressure, you cannot prevent leakage of local up the arm. Choose another technique.

Tom Perris, Gloucester, UK

Difficult i.v. access in a child

Tip

If you have been called by the paediatricians to site a "difficult" i.v. line in a small child, you can bet it is now more difficult as the child has been "Pin cushioned."

Try getting mother and child in the bath together for 15 min. It is not only fun and soothing for the anxious child but provides helpful vasodilation too. First time success and no tears hopefully.

Caveat

For this technique, you need a relatively well child. If he or she is "flat" you just have to get on with it.

Alison Wright, Warwick, UK

Nasogastric tubes

The Surgeons seem to have a habit of announcing they would like an NG tube halfway through the case. The patient then wakes up with an annoying thing down the back of the throat and promptly attempts to pull it out.

The older and more confused patients are, sadly, the ones who probably most need either gastric drainage or enteral nutrition. The need for an NG tube is usually in proportion to the likelihood of it being pulled out.

A few tips to assist with insertion and maintenance.

Tip

When inserting an oral or nasal gastric tube, wrap the last 6 in. Tightly around your fingers. This will create a pigtail twist, which can be used to guide the tube around the curve of the posterior naso/oro pharynx.

Alan B Shang, Duke, USA

Tip

When inserting an NG tube in an intubated patient, move the endotracheal (ET) tube to the far left corner of the mouth.

Using a laryngoscope, sweep the tongue aside as if you were preparing to intubate the trachea but push the "scope" a little further.

With the ET tube out of the way, a clear view of the oesophageal entrance is possible. You can guide the naso-gastric (NG) tube into position with Magill's forceps.

Tom Perris, Gloucester, UK

Tip

If an NG tube is absolutely vital, to reduce the possibility of premature removal, insert one down each nostril. Grasp both tubes with forceps and pull them out of the mouth.

Using a strong, water-resistant tape (Pink "sleek" tape is best) connect the two tubes together so that they are joined in two places either side of the nasal septum.

Tape the distal ends together too ensuring you do not block the holes at the end and reinsert both tubes together down the oesophagus.

It is a rare patient who can pull this out.

To remove, you need to pull the tubes out of the mouth again. Cut the tubes in half, above the join with scissors and, keeping hold of both ends, pull one out the mouth, the other pair out the nose.

It is a bit drastic but it works.

Tom Perris, Gloucester, UK

Tip

When inserting an NG tube, use the curve of the tube to ensure it passes past the soft palate and enters the oropharynx. Now, holding the remainder of the coiled tube in your hand, rotate through 180° so the curve now pushes the tip of the tube against the posterior wall of the pharynx. This reduces the chance of the tube curling forwards and coiling up in the mouth.

Sock Huang Koh, Birmingham, UK

Tip

The correct nostril to choose when inserting an NG tube is the other one. Press the tube against the posterior wall of the pharynx with two fingers and channel it down into the oesophagus.

Failing that, get someone else to do it.

Ben Walton, Bristol, UK

Caveat

If, when asked to empty the stomach during surgery, you aspirate the NG tube and the ventilator starts alarming or the CO_2 trace disappears, you've put it in the lungs not the stomach.

Take it out, re-oxygenate the patient and try again!

Tom Perris, Gloucester, UK

Securing the ET tube

Tip

In patients who have been difficult to intubate or in patients with beards or dirty/oily faces, tape the tube in position and pass the tape circumferentially (behind the patient's neck) and stick it to itself.

This ensures a more secure fixation.

Caveat

Do not occlude the venous return from the head.

Lewis R Hodgins, Duke, USA

Stay dry

Tip

When performing injections for pain relief, (e.g. facet joints, etc.) use a luer-lock syringe to avoid disconnection. The high resistance of the joint capsules makes a "blow-out" likely with consequent loss of injection contents.

Randall P Brewer, Duke, USA

Percutaneous tracheostomy

Tip

Change the ET tube before performing a percutaneous tracheostomy. The more rigid, fresh tube tends not to fall out of the cords so much.

Cannot change the tube? You should not be doing the trachy'!

Also, try using a rigid bronchoscope instead of the fibre-optic scope.

It gives a better picture, is easier to control, holds the trachea more stable and cannot be damaged by the operator's wayward needle.

Jonathan Chantler, Oxford, UK

PRACTICAL PROCEDURES AND TECHNIQUES
Stay dry/Percutaneous tracheostomy

4

CRISIS MANAGEMENT AND EMERGENCIES

I forget who said, "Anaesthesia is 99% boredom and 1% blind panic". It was probably not an anaesthetist as it displays a deal of ignorance about our profession. Most of us do not find our jobs boring and personally, I never let anyone see that I am panicking!

Perhaps it is the 1% moments that make the job so interesting. Conversely, it could be the knowledge that disasters can happen so easily which makes an exemplary anaesthetic so satisfying to administer.

After all, what we do is intrinsically dangerous. Our patients are getting older and sicker, we give them drugs sufficiently toxic to cause unconsciousness, we stop them breathing, we obtund every homeostatic mechanism and safety reflex they possess, and then, we let a surgeon commit grievous bodily harm to them. It is no wonder things sometimes go awry!!

We all get into difficult situations sometimes. Whilst the period of crisis can be exciting, challenging and an opportunity for learning, for the sake of the patient, we should all aim to avoid them if possible. Sometimes that just is not an option.

We include a few tips to remember when the going gets tough.

CRISIS MANAGEMENT AND EMERGENCIES

Tip

No one ever regretted a 14-G intravenous (i.v.) line

Lewis R Hodgins, Duke, USA

In a similar vein (pardon the pun!)

Tip

If you think you might need a big i.v. put in a very big one. If you do not need a big one, use a very small one. Getting stuck in the middle is, on one hand, dangerous and on the other, unnecessarily unpleasant for your patient.

Tom Perris, Gloucester, UK

Tip

If you think to yourself "Might I need a bigger drip?" The answer is "Yes".

In fact, this goes for several things ... should I change the endotracheal (ET) tube? Ring the boss? Write in the notes?

All "Yes".

Ben Walton, Bristol, UK

Tip

In an adult, if all else fails, remember the "Rule of 90s".

- Systolic blood pressure (BP) >90 mmHg.
- Saturation >90%.
- Pulse <90 beats per minute (bpm).

All will be well!

Lewis R Hodgins, Duke, USA

Tip

In cases where all-hell is breaking loose (or you can not explain what is happening) concentrate on the basics of ABC:

Is the airway secure?

Is the patient being ventilated or at least oxygenated?

Do they have a pulse and an end-tidal carbon dioxide (CO_2) trace?

Frequently in the heat of battle I have observed people obsessing with the details (e.g. malfunctioning monitor, kinked i.v. line, etc) only to miss the "important stuff".

Bruce F Cullen, Seattle, WA, USA

Tip

If you know there is trouble on the way, have something to eat and go for a pee. You may not get another chance to perform either of these vital tasks for hours.

Ben Walton, Bristol, UK

Major trauma/emergencies

Tip

If the surgeon is becoming quiet and pale, pay close attention.

Hopefully, your patient is quiet already but may soon be going pale too!

Ben Walton, Bristol, UK

Tip

The sicker your patient, the more the dose of induction agent should be reduced.

Beware of using propofol and particularly thiopentone in patients who are septic or hypovolaemic (or both). Etomidate or ketamine may be a better choice.

Tom Perris, Gloucester, UK

Tip

Where a large volume of fluid is required for restoration of the circulating volume after major trauma, try and ensure that your wide-bore i.v. lines are not sited, so that the fluid you are infusing has to pass the area of trauma to reach the heart.

For example stab wounds to the abdomen or fractured pelvis, site lines in the upper limb, neck or subclavian. Head, chest or upper limb trauma, use the femoral veins.

The reason is this. When the surgeons are attempting to staunch the flow and repair the damage, if, the veins are full of pressurised resuscitation fluid, their view is impeded, the overall blood loss is increased and your precious circulating volume ends up all over the floor.

Caveat

Do not waste time on the niceties of line placement if your patient is about to exsanguinate. Just get the volume in and stop the on-going loss as soon as possible (ASAP). Worry about the rest later.

Tom Perris, Gloucester, UK

Tip

In emergency situations, make sure you are concentrating on the ABCs.

The more unstable the situation, the more need for control of the basics.

Get help for any other tasks that need doing.

Bruce F Cullen, Seattle, WA, USA

Tip

When transfusing blood under pressure, put the blood bags into the infuser with the label facing away from you. When the label is visible through the bag, it is empty.

Ben Walton, Bristol, UK

Anaphylaxis

This is a truly terrifying event if it happens to your patient. Not only are you faced with a rapidly swelling airway, lungs that are impossible to ventilate and a cardiovascular system in collapse but also the knowledge that it was, in all likelihood, you who caused it with your induction agents.

Prompt recognition and action is required. The good news is that simple measures are usually effective.

Tip

In anaphylaxis, the initial dose of epinephrine (adrenaline) is 50 μg i.v. or 300 μg subcutaneously.

Lewis R Hodgins, Duke, USA

Tip

In the event of anaphylaxis, do the obvious:

1. Protect the airway. If not already, intubate the trachea. Give 100% oxygen. Stop giving the drug responsible (if you can identify it).

2. Ventilate the lungs as best you can. Beware of using very high pressures, as pneumothorax is likely. However, you may have no choice.

3. Get (large-bore) i.v. access and give fluid in a hurry. Which particular fluid is unimportant at this point. As long as it is wet and inside the veins it is ok. The only exception is if the fluid is the cause of the anaphylaxis.

4. Give adrenaline. This gets you out of trouble in most cases. Dose titrated to effect (see above tip).

5. Steroids, beta agonists and antihistamines come later. Take blood for tests, etc. later too.

6. Do not stop monitoring the patient once they have improved. Sometimes it comes back.

Tom Perris, Gloucester, UK

Unstable dysrhythmias

Tip

If your patient develops new onset atrial fibrillation (AF), first, try and correct any predisposing cause; hypovolaemia, hypokalaemia and hypomagnesaemia are common culprits.

A 20 mmol of both $MgSO_4$ and KCl and a litre of crystalloid over half an hour is usually about right.

Amiodarone gets you out of nearly all remaining dysrhythmias.

Electricity does the rest.

Tom Perris, Gloucester, UK

Tip

Patients with poorly controlled AF can go rather too fast when reversed with the premixed neostigmine–glycopyrronium.

Try mixing one ampoule of the mixture with one ampoule of plain glycopyrronium.

Discard half of it.

This reduces the proportion of glycopyrronium–neostigmine and results in a slight bradycardia as opposed to a tachycardia.

Much better!

Alastair McCrirrick, Gloucester, UK

Obstetric emergencies

Tip

If you are under pressure from the obstetrician to perform anaesthesia for an emergency caesarean, place your spinal with the patient in lateral position (rather than sitting up).

To my mind, the patient can curl up and open the spaces better (a matter of opinion, I admit) but also, the position of the patient ensures the *heavy Marcain* falls towards the thoracic kyphosis hastening the onset of the block rather than plunging into the sacrum and having to diffuse up again.

Head down tilt speeds onset even more. Needless to say, have a wide-bore i.v. in place and watch the BP carefully.

Tom Perris, Gloucester, UK

Tip

Never anaesthetise a woman of child bearing age with abdominal pain without at least a 16-G i.v. in place.

Ben Walton, Bristol, UK

Tip

Always ask the obstetrician before giving syntocinon.
That way, if there is an unexpected second twin, it is his
fault.

Ben Walton, Bristol, UK

Tip

If the patient is losing blood, syntocinon is your first resort to
contract the uterus and compress the bleeding vessels.
Do not give more that 5 IU as a bolus. It causes vasodilation
and can precipitate cardiovascular collapse in the presence
of hypovolaemia. If you need more, start an infusion or use
something else.

Ergometrine is your next line. Failing that, get the surgeon to
inject prostaglandin ("haemabate") into the uterus.

Sock Huang Koh, Birmingham, UK

Bronchospasm

Tip

If the patient develops bronchospasm, a dose of beta agonist
can be delivered into the circuit via the angled connector.

Connect a 50 mL luer-lock syringe to the capnography port.
Drop a salbutamol inhaler into the barrel and use the
plunger to spray the drug into the airway during inspiration.

Alastair McCrirrick, Gloucester, UK

Tip

Bronchospasm in intubated patients is often due to irritation of the carina. Try pulling the tube back a centimetre or two. Try increasing the inspired agent too.

Tom Perris, Gloucester, UK

Decision-making

It is easy to start something. It is harder to stop. Think carefully before embarking on an action that may not be in the best interests of the patient.

Tip

If the patient is moribund or approaching it, remember this: the best anaesthetic for this patient may be no anaesthetic. Death is inevitable eventually. The patient should not be denied a "good" end to their life by unnecessary intervention. Do not use technology to prolong death. Use it to enhance life.

Ben Walton, Bristol, UK

5

MISCELLANEOUS

We received many tips from many contributors. Not all of them were printable but we have included the majority. Several of the suggestions did not fit easily into a category so we have included a miscellany of this advice. We like to think there is at least a shred of wisdom in all the tips we have shared with you. Well, some of them are funny anyway!

> **Tip**
>
> Never start a case until you see the whites of the surgeon's eyes, in theatre. Even BMWs get stuck in traffic.
>
> *Ben Walton, Bristol, UK*

Securing intravenous lines

> **Tip**
>
> Tape all your drips in well (or sew them). Keep all giving sets untangled and take great care on moving or transferring the patient. Disconnect everything possible before moving. It is a pain but not so much as replacing all your lines or the endotracheal (ET) tube.
>
> *Tom Perris, Gloucester, UK*

"Stay humble"

A venerable consultant told me this on my first day as an Anaesthetic Senior House Officer (SHO). I have always tried to follow his advice. I pass it on to you.

Tip

You will make mistakes in your career. Gradually these will get less and your confidence will increase. Whatever you do, "stay humble." The minute you start to think you can do anything, anaesthesia will bite you in the arse!

Wise words!

Tom Perris, Gloucester, UK

Physics

Tip

Physics teaches us many things applicable to anaesthesia. The study of hydraulics says that force over area equals pressure. This is why that clotted cannula you have struggled to insert can be cleared effectively with a 2 mL syringe rather than a 10 mL. Same force, smaller area and higher pressure.

That is the reason why there is so much of it in the examination syllabus.

Ben Walton, Bristol, UK

Tip

If you find that a fine bore nasogastric (NG) feeding tube has become blocked, 2 mL of Coca Cola squirted down it will reliably clear the blockage. The small syringe provides high pressure and the corrosive properties of coke do the rest.

Kay Chidley, Gloucester, UK

> **Tip**
>
> Put a long loop of your drip tubing inside the hose of the warming blanket. You get a free fluid warmer.
>
> *Jonathan Chantler, Oxford, UK*

> **Tip**
>
> If you have to place your intravenous (i.v.) in the same arm as the blood pressure (BP) cuff, try putting a loop of the giving set under the cuff. Then, when the cuff inflates, the drip is temporarily kinked and the drip does not bleed back into the line.
>
> *Kay Chidley, Gloucester, UK*

Operating lights

> **Tip**
>
> An operating light shone straight on to an Ohmeda flow sensor will disable it and a low-tidal volume alarm will sound.
>
> Move the light.
>
> *Lewis R Hodgins, Duke, USA*

Vasodilation after cardiopulmonary bypass

> **Tip**
>
> There is often a problem with persistent vasodilation after a long cardiopulmonary bypass (CPB) time especially if cell salvage was used.

High-dose steroids (e.g. 1 G solumedrol) may rectify the situation.

Lewis R Hodgins, Duke, USA

Labour ward politics

The person who supplied this one wanted to remain anonymous. The authors do not necessarily concur with its sentiments. We include it for completeness.

Tip

Never argue with a midwife.

They have no interest in what you have to say and would not understand it if they had.

Save your breath.

Anonymous Obstetric Anaesthetist, London, UK

Topical local anaesthetic

Tip

Never offer to demonstrate how quickly topical anaesthesia works by applying it to your tongue. It taste revolting and makes your mouth go all funny.

Get the trainee to do it on himself.

Ben Walton, Bristol, UK

I was told this one by someone who is now very senior indeed in the Royal College of Anaesthetists (London).

> **Tip**
>
> The only reason, ever, to adjust a surgeon's light for him is to turn it off until someone competent comes to stand underneath it.
>
> *Tom Perris, Gloucester, UK*

The bigger they are ...

> **Tip**
>
> Never stick a needle into anyone over 6 ft tall or 100 kg in weight unless they are lying down, especially if they say they will be fine.
>
> Likewise, never let a man watch his operation under regional anaesthesia.
>
> *Ben Walton, Bristol, UK*

Gloves

> **Tip**
>
> Do not attempt to handle any sort of adhesive tape when wearing latex gloves. Unless you want to amuse your colleagues.
>
> *Tom Perris, Gloucester, UK*

Tip

Stick two pieces of eye tape to the face mask before induction. They will be conveniently located so you can protect the eyes before inserting the ET tube.

Scott Brudney, Duke, USA

Colleagues

Tip

If a member of staff is having treatment, the chances of a complication are proportional to the seniority of the colleague.

If you are the member of staff (and all goes well) remember to thank the entire theatre team. Very few anaesthetists will be offended by a decent bottle of wine.

Tom Perris, Gloucester, UK

Printed in the United States
by Baker & Taylor Publisher Services